30 days to Making Health a Habit

And your time starts NOW

Date:

_____

My Monthly Food Journal

Good food is an important part of a balanced diet.

There is a saying - you can't manage what you don't measure.

Measuring your intake helps you manage your output.

A healthier inside makes for a more attractive outside.

Become your own Boss today, by managing what you eat, and how you use those calories

Habit Tracker

Month _____

Year _____

Day

Day															
1															
2															
3															
4															
5															
6															
7															
8															
9															
10															
11															
12															
13															
14															
15															
16															
17															
18															
19															
20															
21															
22															
23															
24															
25															
26															
27															
28															
29															
30															
31															

Notes:

Date		S M T W T F S
Breakfast	Amount	Calories (kcal)
	Total	
Snack	Amount	Calories (kcal)
	Total	
Lunch	Amount	Calories (kcal)
	Total	

Snack	Amount	Calories (kcal)
	Total	

Dinner	Amount	Calories (kcal)
	Total	

Snack	Amount	Calories (kcal)
	Total	

Exercise	Duration	Calories burned (kcal)

Water							Fruit & Veggies						

Notes:

Date		S M T W T F S
Breakfast	Amount	Calories (kcal)
	Total	
Snack	Amount	Calories (kcal)
	Total	
Lunch	Amount	Calories (kcal)
	Total	

Snack	Amount	Calories (kcal)
	Total	
Dinner	Amount	Calories (kcal)
	Total	
Snack	Amount	Calories (kcal)
	Total	
Exercise	Duration	Calories burned (kcal)
Water	Fruit & Veggies	

Notes:

Date		S M T W T F S
Breakfast	Amount	Calories (kcal)
	Total	
Snack	Amount	Calories (kcal)
	Total	
Lunch	Amount	Calories (kcal)
	Total	

Snack	Amount	Calories (kcal)
	Total	
Dinner	Amount	Calories (kcal)
	Total	
Snack	Amount	Calories (kcal)
	Total	
Exercise	Duration	Calories burned (kcal)
Water		Fruit & Veggies	

Notes:

Date		S M T W T F S	
Breakfast	Amount	Calories (kcal)	
	Total		
Snack	Amount	Calories (kcal)	
	Total		
Lunch	Amount	Calories (kcal)	
	Total		

Snack	Amount	Calories (kcal)
	Total	
Dinner	Amount	Calories (kcal)
	Total	
Snack	Amount	Calories (kcal)
	Total	
Exercise	Duration	Calories burned (kcal)
Water		Fruit & Veggies

Notes:

Date	S M T W T F S	
Breakfast	Amount	Calories (kcal)
	Total	
Snack	Amount	Calories (kcal)
	Total	
Lunch	Amount	Calories (kcal)
	Total	

Snack	Amount	Calories (kcal)
	Total	
Dinner	Amount	Calories (kcal)
	Total	
Snack	Amount	Calories (kcal)
	Total	
Exercise	Duration	Calories burned (kcal)
Water	Fruit & Veggies	

Notes:

Date	S M T W T F S	
Breakfast	Amount	Calories (kcal)
	Total	
Snack	Amount	Calories (kcal)
	Total	
Lunch	Amount	Calories (kcal)
	Total	

Snack	Amount	Calories (kcal)
	Total	
Dinner	Amount	Calories (kcal)
	Total	
Snack	Amount	Calories (kcal)
	Total	
Exercise	Duration	Calories burned (kcal)
Water		Fruit & Veggies	

Notes:

Date	S M T W T F S	
Breakfast	Amount	Calories (kcal)
	Total	
Snack	Amount	Calories (kcal)
	Total	
Lunch	Amount	Calories (kcal)
	Total	

Snack	Amount	Calories (kcal)
	Total	
Dinner	Amount	Calories (kcal)
	Total	
Snack	Amount	Calories (kcal)
	Total	
Exercise	Duration	Calories burned (kcal)
Water	Fruit & Veggies	

Notes:

Date		S M T W T F S
Breakfast	Amount	Calories (kcal)
	Total	
Snack	Amount	Calories (kcal)
	Total	
Lunch	Amount	Calories (kcal)
	Total	

Snack	Amount	Calories (kcal)
	Total	
Dinner	Amount	Calories (kcal)
	Total	
Snack	Amount	Calories (kcal)
	Total	
Exercise	Duration	Calories burned (kcal)
Water	Fruit & Veggies	

Notes:

Date		S M T W T F S	
Breakfast		Amount	Calories (kcal)
		Total	
Snack		Amount	Calories (kcal)
		Total	
Lunch		Amount	Calories (kcal)
		Total	

Snack	Amount	Calories (kcal)
	Total	

Dinner	Amount	Calories (kcal)
	Total	

Snack	Amount	Calories (kcal)
	Total	

Exercise	Duration	Calories burned (kcal)

Water								Fruit & Veggies							

Notes:

Date		S M T W T F S
Breakfast	Amount	Calories (kcal)
	Total	
Snack	Amount	Calories (kcal)
	Total	
Lunch	Amount	Calories (kcal)
	Total	

Snack	Amount	Calories (kcal)
	Total	
Dinner	Amount	Calories (kcal)
	Total	
Snack	Amount	Calories (kcal)
	Total	
Exercise	Duration	Calories burned (kcal)
Water	Fruit & Veggies	

Notes:

Date	S M T W T F S	
Breakfast	Amount	Calories (kcal)
	Total	
Snack	Amount	Calories (kcal)
	Total	
Lunch	Amount	Calories (kcal)
	Total	

Snack	Amount	Calories (kcal)
	Total	
Dinner	Amount	Calories (kcal)
	Total	
Snack	Amount	Calories (kcal)
	Total	
Exercise	Duration	Calories burned (kcal)
Water		Fruit & Veggies

Notes:

Date		S M T W T F S
Breakfast	Amount	Calories (kcal)
	Total	
Snack	Amount	Calories (kcal)
	Total	
Lunch	Amount	Calories (kcal)
	Total	

Snack	Amount	Calories (kcal)
	Total	
Dinner	Amount	Calories (kcal)
	Total	
Snack	Amount	Calories (kcal)
	Total	
Exercise	Duration	Calories burned (kcal)
Water	Fruit & Veggies	

Notes:

Date		S M T W T F S	
Breakfast	Amount	Calories (kcal)	
	Total		
Snack	Amount	Calories (kcal)	
	Total		
Lunch	Amount	Calories (kcal)	
	Total		

Snack	Amount	Calories (kcal)
	Total	
Dinner	Amount	Calories (kcal)
	Total	
Snack	Amount	Calories (kcal)
	Total	
Exercise	Duration	Calories burned (kcal)
Water	Fruit & Veggies	

Notes:

Date		S M T W T F S	
Breakfast	Amount		Calories (kcal)
	Total		
Snack	Amount		Calories (kcal)
	Total		
Lunch	Amount		Calories (kcal)
	Total		

Snack	Amount	Calories (kcal)
	Total	
Dinner	Amount	Calories (kcal)
	Total	
Snack	Amount	Calories (kcal)
	Total	
Exercise	Duration	Calories burned (kcal)
Water		Fruit & Veggies

Notes:

Date	S M T W T F S	
Breakfast	Amount	Calories (kcal)
	Total	
Snack	Amount	Calories (kcal)
	Total	
Lunch	Amount	Calories (kcal)
	Total	

Snack	Amount	Calories (kcal)
	Total	
Dinner	Amount	Calories (kcal)
	Total	
Snack	Amount	Calories (kcal)
	Total	
Exercise	Duration	Calories burned (kcal)
Water	Fruit & Veggies	

Notes:

Date		S M T W T F S
Breakfast	Amount	Calories (kcal)
	Total	
Snack	Amount	Calories (kcal)
	Total	
Lunch	Amount	Calories (kcal)
	Total	

Snack	Amount	Calories (kcal)
	Total	
Dinner	Amount	Calories (kcal)
	Total	
Snack	Amount	Calories (kcal)
	Total	
Exercise	Duration	Calories burned (kcal)
Water	Fruit & Veggies	

Notes:

Date		S M T W T F S	
Breakfast		Amount	Calories (kcal)
		Total	
Snack		Amount	Calories (kcal)
		Total	
Lunch		Amount	Calories (kcal)
		Total	

Snack	Amount	Calories (kcal)
	Total	

Dinner	Amount	Calories (kcal)
	Total	

Snack	Amount	Calories (kcal)
	Total	

Exercise	Duration	Calories burned (kcal)

Water		Fruit & Veggies	

Notes:

Date		S M T W T F S	
Breakfast	Amount		Calories (kcal)
	Total		
Snack	Amount		Calories (kcal)
	Total		
Lunch	Amount		Calories (kcal)
	Total		

Snack	Amount	Calories (kcal)
	Total	
Dinner	Amount	Calories (kcal)
	Total	
Snack	Amount	Calories (kcal)
	Total	
Exercise	Duration	Calories burned (kcal)
Water								Fruit & Veggies						

Notes:

Date		S M T W T F S	
Breakfast		Amount	Calories (kcal)
		Total	
Snack		Amount	Calories (kcal)
		Total	
Lunch		Amount	Calories (kcal)
		Total	

Snack	Amount	Calories (kcal)
	Total	

Dinner	Amount	Calories (kcal)
	Total	

Snack	Amount	Calories (kcal)
	Total	

Exercise	Duration	Calories burned (kcal)

Water		Fruit & Veggies	

Notes:

Date	S M T W T F S	
Breakfast	Amount	Calories (kcal)
	Total	
Snack	Amount	Calories (kcal)
	Total	
Lunch	Amount	Calories (kcal)
	Total	

Snack	Amount	Calories (kcal)
	Total	
Dinner	Amount	Calories (kcal)
	Total	
Snack	Amount	Calories (kcal)
	Total	
Exercise	Duration	Calories burned (kcal)
Water		Fruit & Veggies

Notes:

Date	S M T W T F S	
Breakfast	Amount	Calories (kcal)
	Total	
Snack	Amount	Calories (kcal)
	Total	
Lunch	Amount	Calories (kcal)
	Total	

Snack	Amount	Calories (kcal)
	Total	
Dinner	Amount	Calories (kcal)
	Total	
Snack	Amount	Calories (kcal)
	Total	
Exercise	Duration	Calories burned (kcal)

Water								Fruit & Veggies							

Notes:

Date		S M T W T F S	
Breakfast		Amount	Calories (kcal)
		Total	
Snack		Amount	Calories (kcal)
		Total	
Lunch		Amount	Calories (kcal)
		Total	

Snack	Amount	Calories (kcal)
	Total	
Dinner	Amount	Calories (kcal)
	Total	
Snack	Amount	Calories (kcal)
	Total	
Exercise	Duration	Calories burned (kcal)
Water		Fruit & Veggies

Notes:

Date		S M T W T F S
Breakfast	Amount	Calories (kcal)
	Total	
Snack	Amount	Calories (kcal)
	Total	
Lunch	Amount	Calories (kcal)
	Total	

Snack	Amount	Calories (kcal)
	Total	
Dinner	Amount	Calories (kcal)
	Total	
Snack	Amount	Calories (kcal)
	Total	
Exercise	Duration	Calories burned (kcal)

Water								Fruit & Veggies								

Notes:

Date		S M T W T F S
Breakfast	Amount	Calories (kcal)
	Total	
Snack	Amount	Calories (kcal)
	Total	
Lunch	Amount	Calories (kcal)
	Total	

Snack	Amount	Calories (kcal)
	Total	
Dinner	Amount	Calories (kcal)
	Total	
Snack	Amount	Calories (kcal)
	Total	
Exercise	Duration	Calories burned (kcal)
Water		Fruit & Veggies	

Notes:

Date		S M T W T F S
Breakfast	Amount	Calories (kcal)
	Total	
Snack	Amount	Calories (kcal)
	Total	
Lunch	Amount	Calories (kcal)
	Total	

Snack	Amount	Calories (kcal)
	Total	

Dinner	Amount	Calories (kcal)
	Total	

Snack	Amount	Calories (kcal)
	Total	

Exercise	Duration	Calories burned (kcal)

Water									Fruit & Veggies								

Notes:

Date		S M T W T F S	
Breakfast	Amount		Calories (kcal)
	Total		
Snack	Amount		Calories (kcal)
	Total		
Lunch	Amount		Calories (kcal)
	Total		

Snack	Amount	Calories (kcal)
	Total	
Dinner	Amount	Calories (kcal)
	Total	
Snack	Amount	Calories (kcal)
	Total	
Exercise	Duration	Calories burned (kcal)
Water		Fruit & Veggies

Notes:

Date		S M T W T F S
Breakfast	Amount	Calories (kcal)
	Total	
Snack	Amount	Calories (kcal)
	Total	
Lunch	Amount	Calories (kcal)
	Total	

Snack	Amount	Calories (kcal)
	Total	

Dinner	Amount	Calories (kcal)
	Total	

Snack	Amount	Calories (kcal)
	Total	

Exercise	Duration	Calories burned (kcal)

Water								Fruit & Veggies							

Notes:

Date		S M T W T F S	
Breakfast		Amount	Calories (kcal)
		Total	
Snack		Amount	Calories (kcal)
		Total	
Lunch		Amount	Calories (kcal)
		Total	

Snack	Amount	Calories (kcal)
	Total	
Dinner	Amount	Calories (kcal)
	Total	
Snack	Amount	Calories (kcal)
	Total	
Exercise	Duration	Calories burned (kcal)
Water									Fruit & Veggies							

Notes:

Date		S M T W T F S	
Breakfast		Amount	Calories (kcal)
		Total	
Snack		Amount	Calories (kcal)
		Total	
Lunch		Amount	Calories (kcal)
		Total	

Snack	Amount	Calories (kcal)
	Total	
Dinner	Amount	Calories (kcal)
	Total	
Snack	Amount	Calories (kcal)
	Total	
Exercise	Duration	Calories burned (kcal)
Water	Fruit & Veggies	

Notes:

Date		S M T W T F S	
Breakfast	Amount		Calories (kcal)
	Total		
Snack	Amount		Calories (kcal)
	Total		
Lunch	Amount		Calories (kcal)
	Total		

Snack	Amount	Calories (kcal)
	Total	
Dinner	Amount	Calories (kcal)
	Total	
Snack	Amount	Calories (kcal)
	Total	
Exercise	Duration	Calories burned (kcal)
Water		Fruit & Veggies	

Notes:

Notes: